Your Beautiful Birth

Workbook

By April Wood

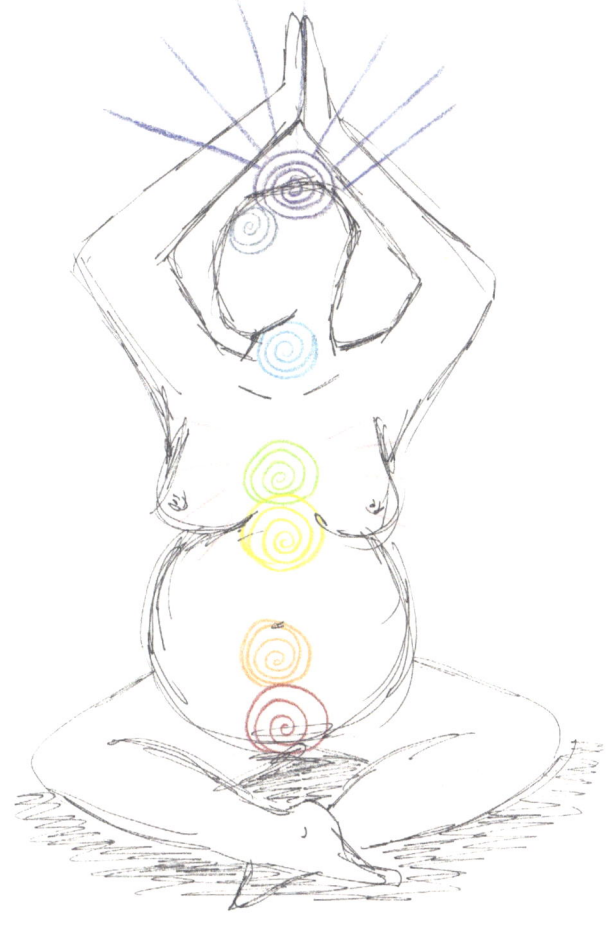

Introduction

First of all before you go any further-

Congratulations on your pregnancy!

This workbook is designed to help you sit down and focus on what you want through your birth. Birth is such a personal experience, it is so easy to get caught up in what everyone else wants- now is the time to sit down and work out what you want.

It is designed not to provide you with all of your options, or information, but more to prompt your thinking, encourage you to explore those options and then write them down so that you can focus on making them a reality.

A great birth isn't a coincidence, most of the time it is the women who are empowered with knowledge, who have done the work before hand that have a positive birth experience.

Take your time working through this book, birth isn't a process to be rushed or shrugged off. Birth is a transformative experience that can have impact on all areas of your life. Take the time to honor that and respect the importance of that.

You can do this, and you can do this beautifully!

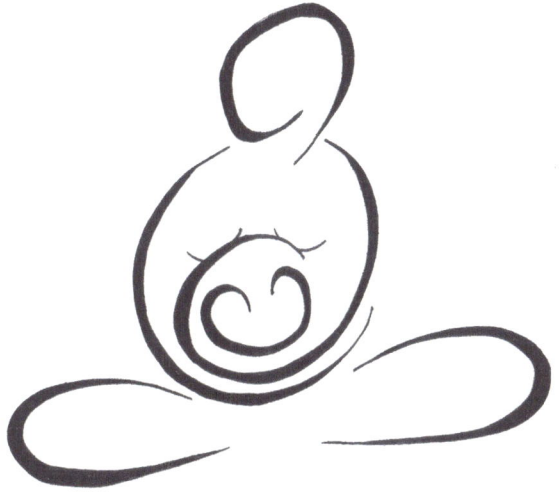

The idea behind this eBook, is that you print it out, and fill it in. You will then be able to keep it as a part of your journey, and later pass it on to your child as a momento of the path you took bringing them into the world.

In doing this you will be able to omit or duplicate pages to suit your own needs. For example you might need 4 pages to complete your birth story after your baby is born, or some of the pages may not be relevant to you (such as if this is your first birth, the pages regarding your other births won't apply). Please note that page 30 is intentionally blank so please feel free to print as many times as needed if extra room required.

Remember that there is no "right" or "wrong" way of filling in this book, it is your book, so you fill it in how you want. You might want to draw, you might want to write, you might want to create a collage!

Just make sure you are honest with yourself, and answer truthfully, from the heart. Have fun with this book, take your time, make it something that you are proud of, that you are consciously creating.

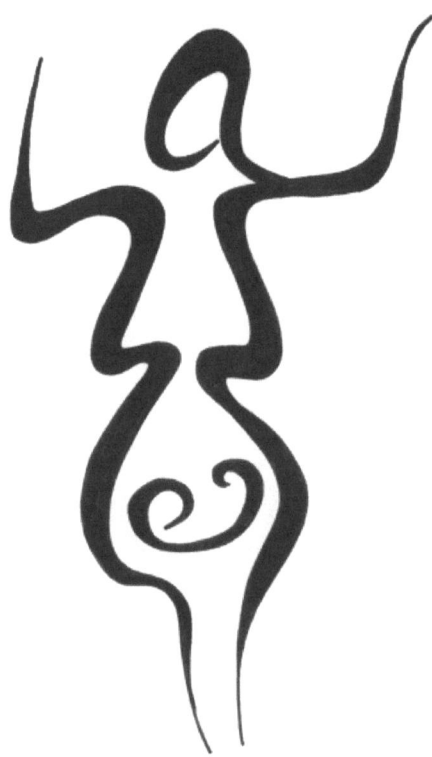

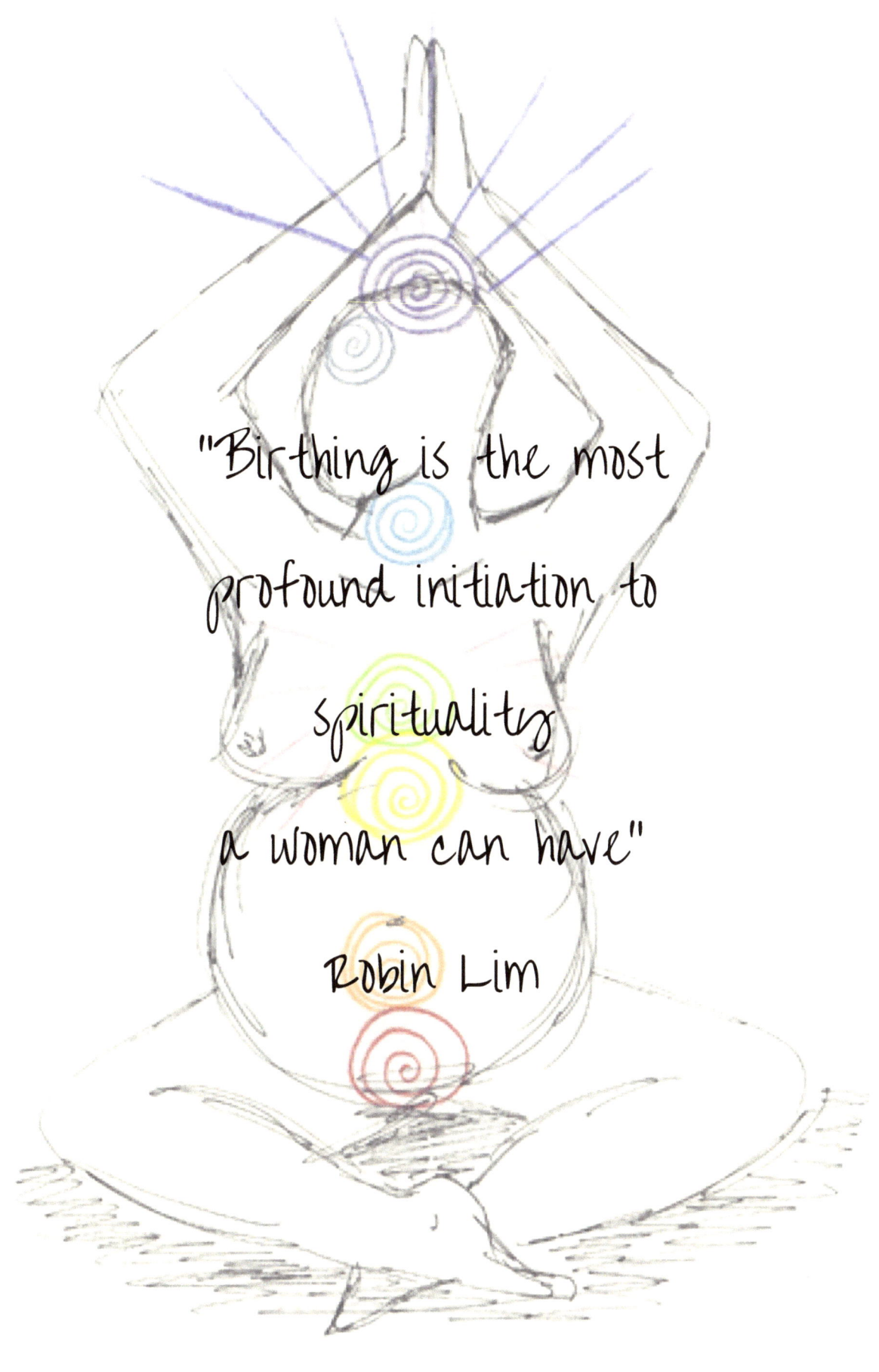

"Birthing is the most profound initiation to spirituality a woman can have"

Robin Lim

what are the top 3 goals for your birth?

Birth goals are important to help you identify what are the most important aspects of the birth are for you. For some women they may include feeling as little pain as possible, for others it may be to have a natural, drug free vaginal birth. By setting out your birth goals at the start of this workbook, it will help you to assess whether your choices throughout the rest of the book are aligned with these goals or not. Then you will be able to adjust either your goals, or choices along the way.

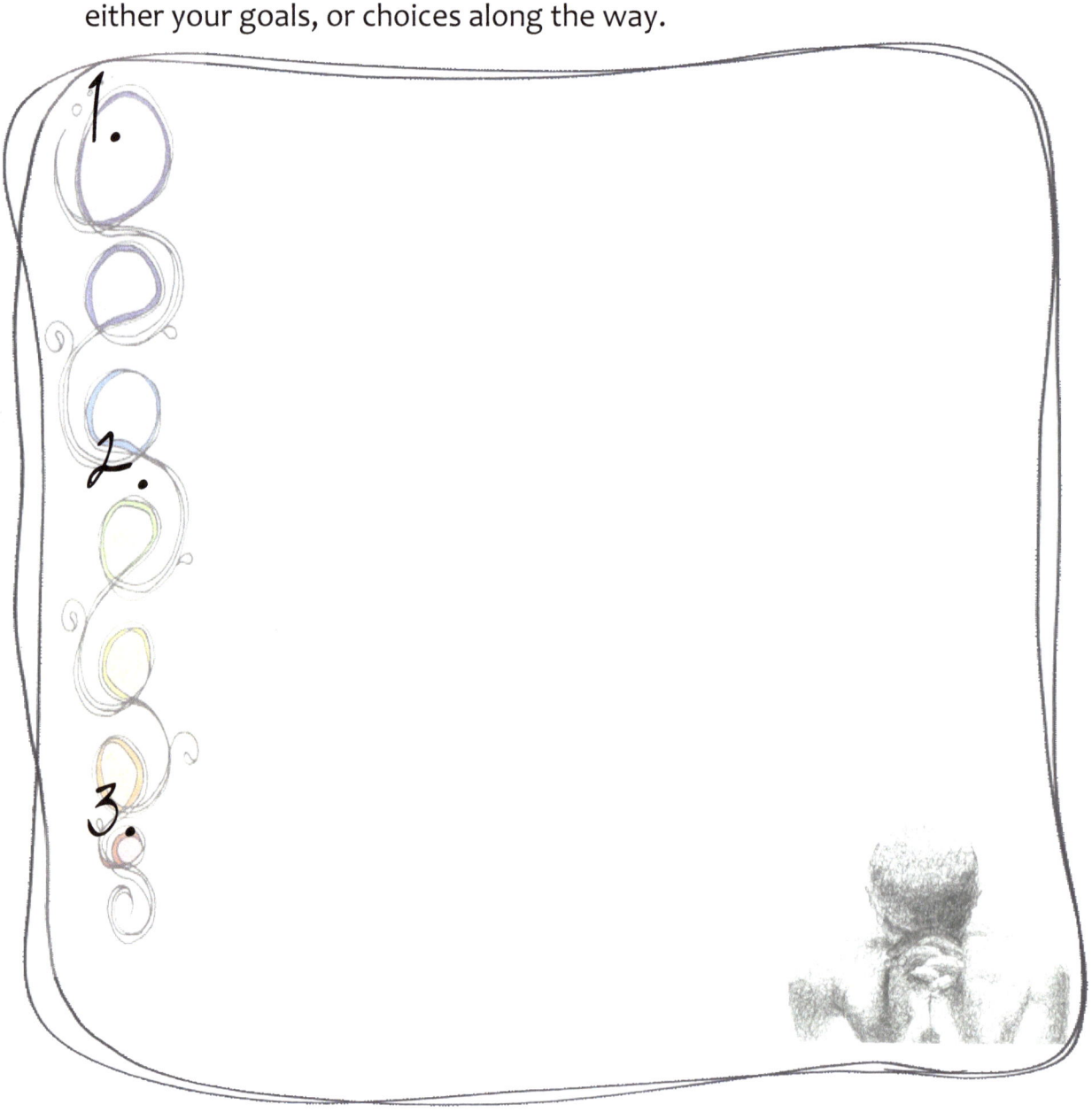

1.

2.

3.

what did you love about your last birth?

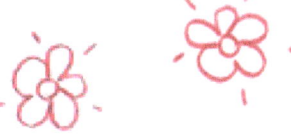

It is important to sit back and think about our previous births, so that we are able to learn from our mistakes. Take some time to think about what you loved about your last birth, what will you do again?

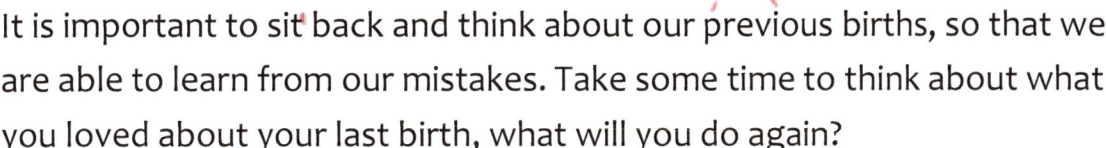

what would you change about your last birth?

Similarly, it is important to recognize what we can do differently if we had an experience that we may not have liked. Take some time to think about what decisions you can make differently this time to help change the outcome. Remember, the more involvement you have in your care, the more power you have, and thus the more empowerment and satisfaction.

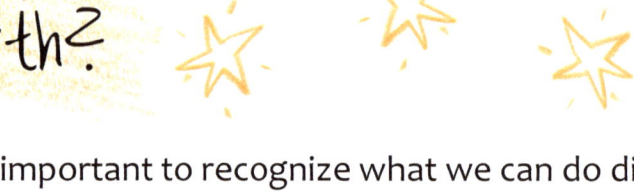

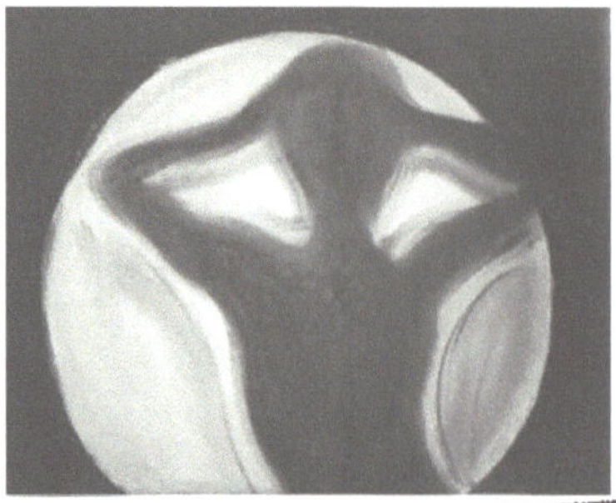

who would you like at your birth?

Your care provider is of the utmost importance when it comes to birth- even more so than where you give birth. If your ideals and philosophy don't match with your care providers, it may make your goals unrealistic, which can then lead on to feelings of dissatisfaction or trauma.

Remember that it is NEVER too late to change your care provider (even if you are in labour!)

Other than your care provide, who else would you like to be there? How would you like them to support you?

"If I don't know
my options,
I don't have any."

Diana Korte

who are your support people?

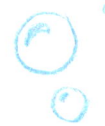

This is different to your care provider. Your care provider will be helping you in a medical capacity, a support person is there to support you in an emotional capacity.

Who would you like to have there to support you emotionally? Common choices are: mother, best friend or doula.

Take some time to think about how you would like to be supported, and ideally what tasks you would like your support people to carry out. Make sure you sit down and talk to them about it, so that everyone knows what your expectations are.

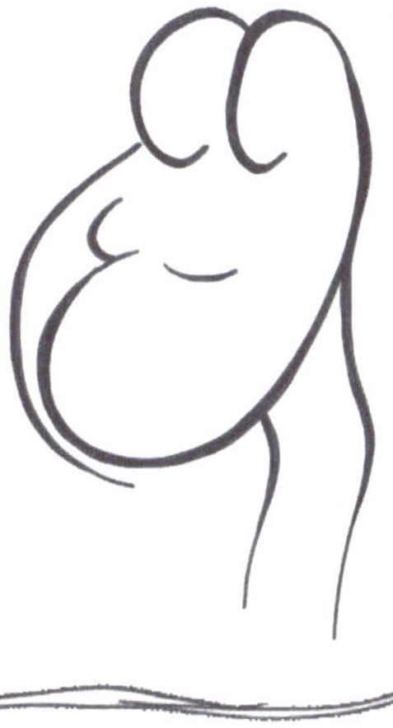

where would you like to give birth?

Once you know who your care provider is, you will likely know where you are going to give birth. Common choices are: hospital, birthing centre, or at home. Each location will have its own benefits, and disadvantages- it is up to you to ensure you make the choice that is most appropriate to you and your family.

Take some time to think about how you might be able to make the location as comfortable as you can.

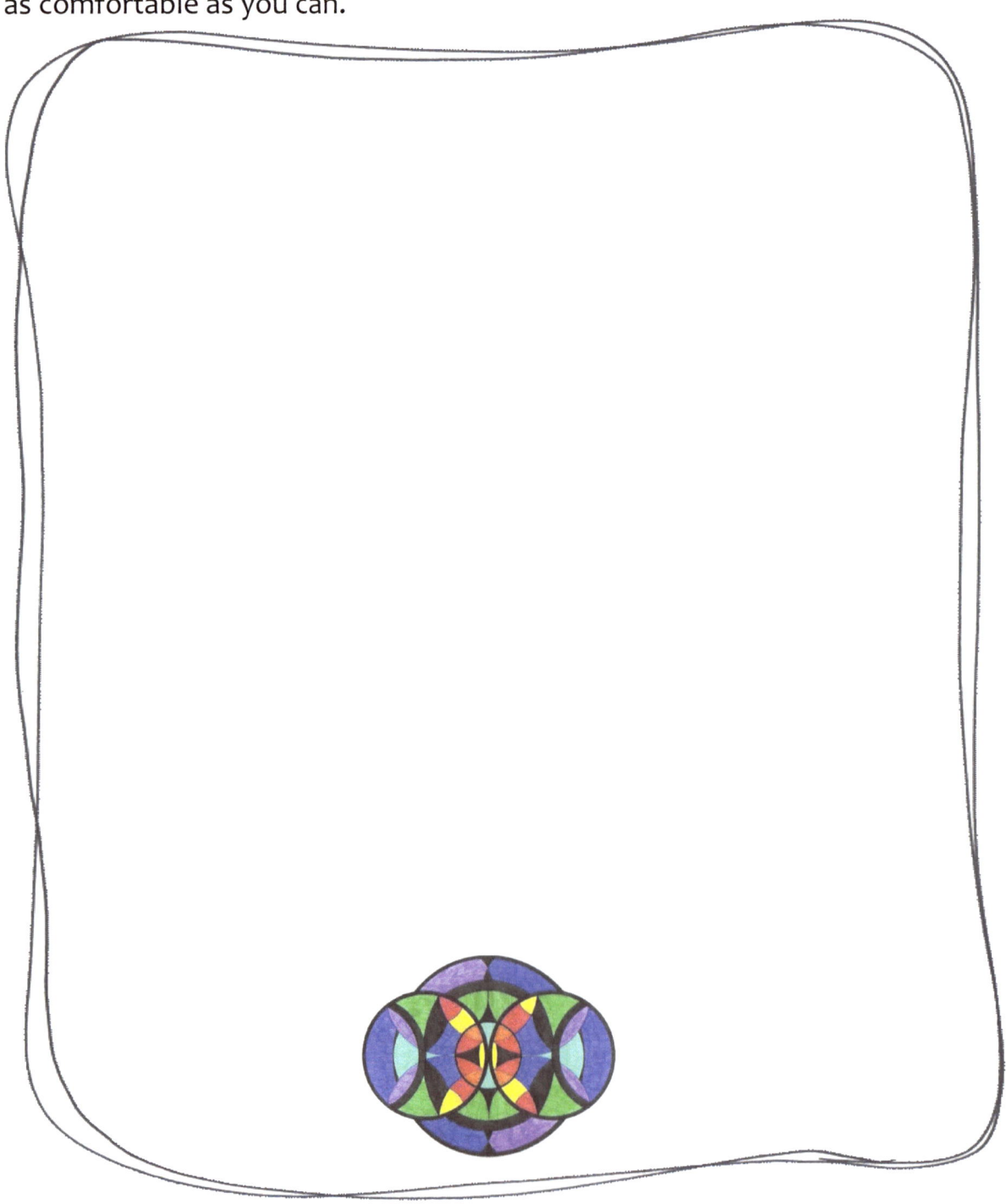

what are three things that give you strength?

Often in birth women reach a point of "I just can't do this" it is no reflection on the woman, or her ability to birth. Some say that it is the passage of maiden to mother.

It is great to be prepared, and to know what gives you strength, so that when you are in labour you will be able to draw on those things to help you get through and achieve your goals.

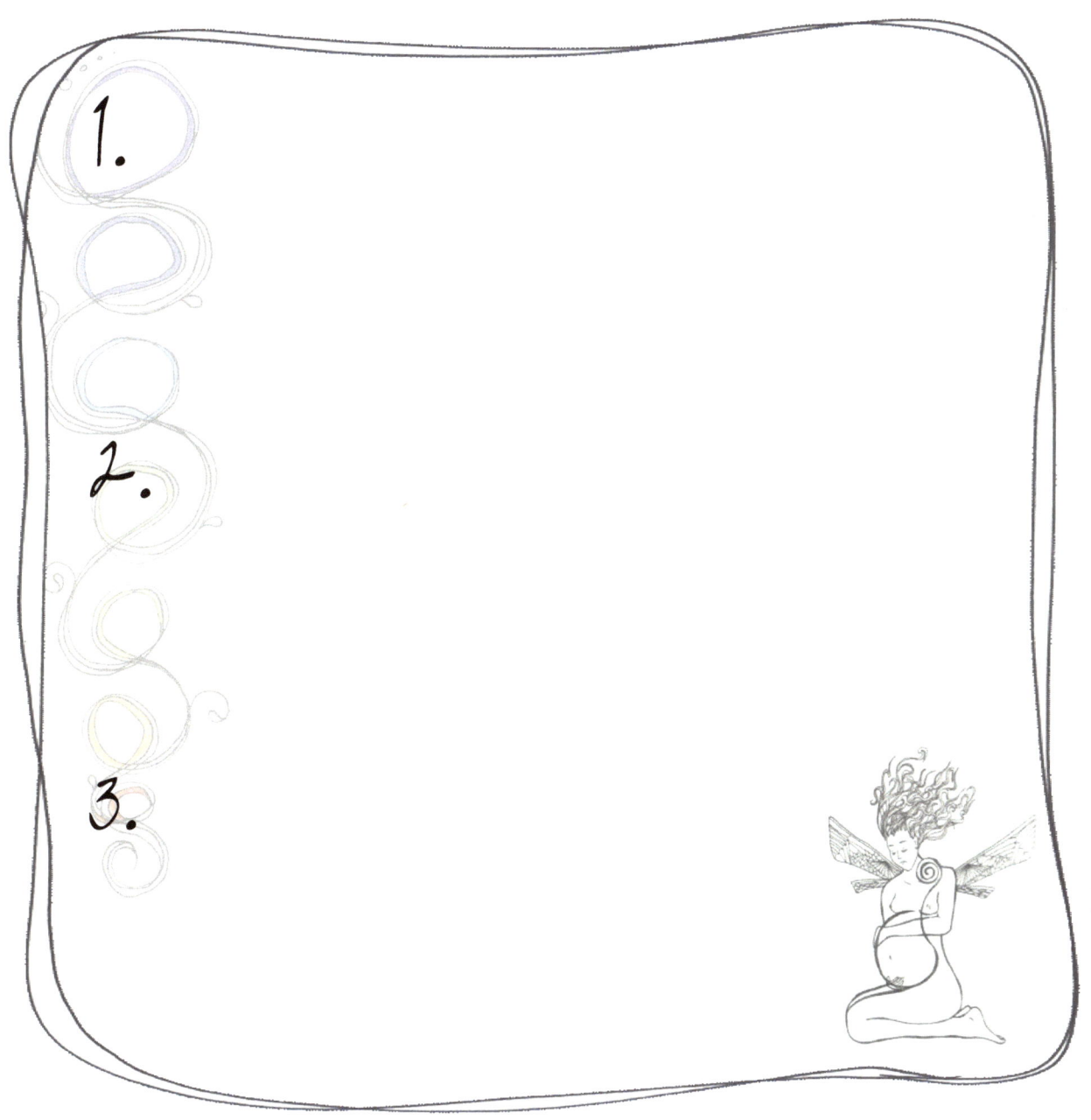

1.

2.

3.

"The knowledge of how to give birth without outside interventions lies deep within each woman"

unknown

what are your fears?

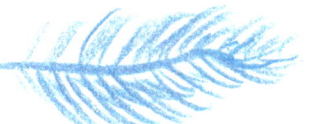

When we are in labour, if we have fears, or emotional blockages it can cause our birth to slow down, stop, or sometimes not start at all!
It is recommended to explore any fears that you have while you are pregnant, this will help you to recognise any potential issues, and allow you to raise them with your care provider and support people. It doesn't matter how silly a fear might seem- if it is a reality to you it is worth looking into and exploring.

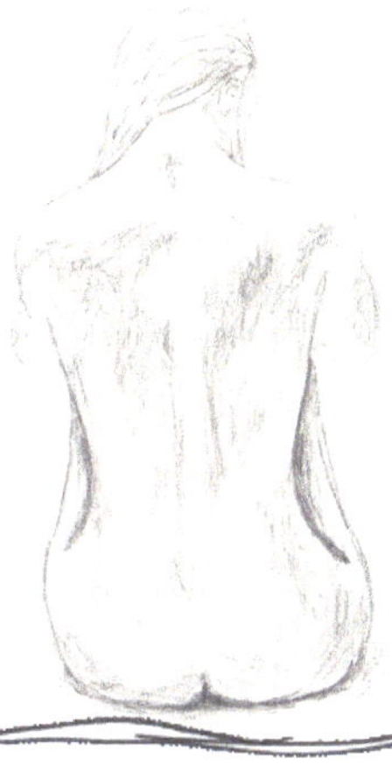

what images come to mind with birth?

The images that come to mind when we think about birthing are important, they help to provide us insight into how our subconscious feels about birth. The way birth is portrayed in the media is generally not an accurate depiction; there is a lot of negativity and fear. Birth is empowering, inspiring, beautiful and a time of growth. To change your way of thinking start sourcing books, or watching movies of empowering births, and surround yourself with positive birth stories.

what pain relief are you planning to use?

There are many methods of pain relief to use in labour. Some of them are medical, but many more are natural and non-pharmaceutical. The benefits of non-medical pain relief are that there are no side effects for your baby, and generally less/none for you too. Some examples are heat, water, massage, meditation, or music. What are some of the ways you would like to manage the pain experienced during birth?

"The power and intensity
of your contractions
cannot be stronger than you,
because it is you."

Unknown

what music do you want to listen to?

Some women find it comforting, and relaxing to listen to music while they are in labour. If listened to using headphones it can be a great tool to help you focus within, and remove any distractions.

what images would you like to look at?

Images or pictures can work wonderfully as a focus point during labour. Have a think about what images bring you joy, happiness or represent birth to you. Try to keep them positive, and make copies of the images to have with you when you birth to draw strength from.

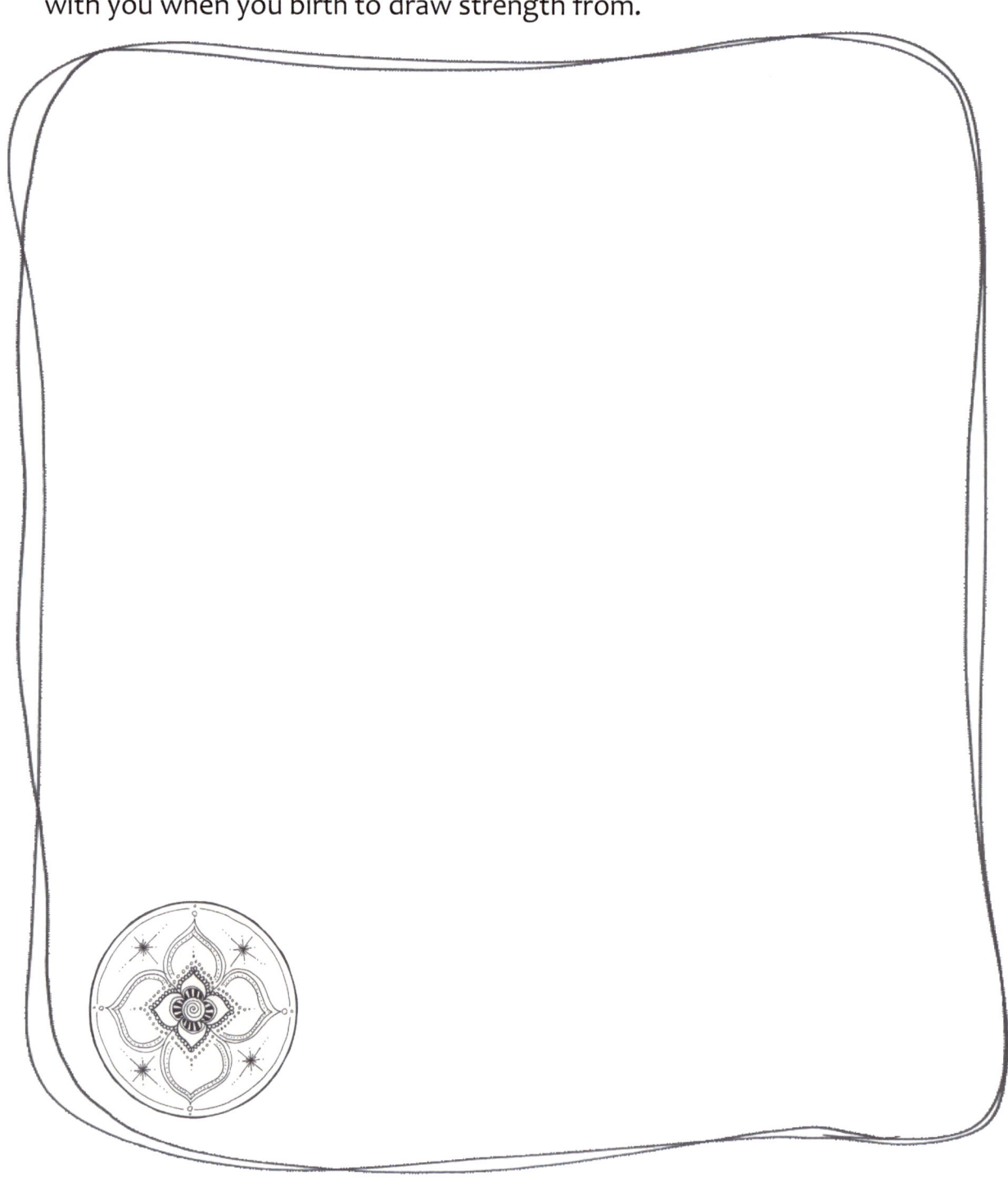

Planning a caesarean?

You may feel like you have limited choices when you have a planned caesarean. In fact this is not true at all! The benefit of planning a caesarean is that you have the ability to plan ahead, and talk to your care provider about what your expectations are. For some ideas you can google "natural caesarean" and see what information comes up.

what about unexpected situations?

It is important to consider what you and your support people may do in the event of unexpected situations. Will you want to consider all of your options before making decisions? If you and the baby need to be separated, who will stay with you, who will stay with the baby? What is your back up if your birth doesn't go according to plan?

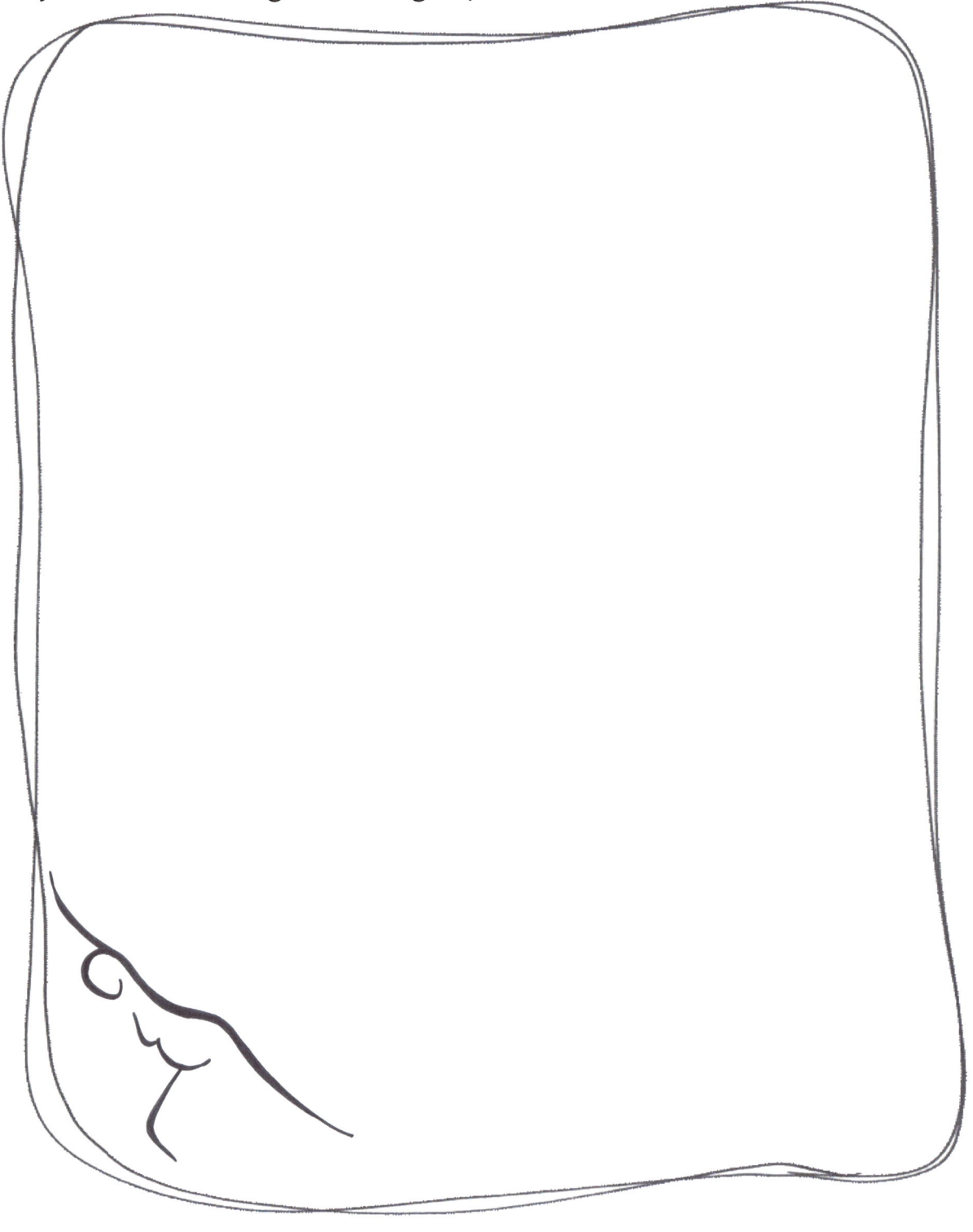

"Giving birth should be
your greatest achievement
not your greatest fear."

Jane Weideman

Immediately after the birth

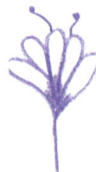

Straight after you have birthed your baby is a very important time for you and your baby's bonding. Close your eyes and have a think about how you imagine the first 10 minutes of your baby's life earthside, what does this look like? Keep in mind that many of the routine checks and tests are able to wait.

your placenta options

Immediately after the birth, you will need to birth your placenta. There are different options you can choose- whether you want to let your body do it naturally, or have medication to assist.

There are also choices regarding what you would like to do with the placenta afterwards. Some women choose to take it home and bury it under a tree, some choose to consume it, some encapsulate it. If you are wanting to take your placenta home (if you are not birthing at home), it is important to make this clear to your care providers, as it is typically incinerated as medical waste.

How will you feed your baby?

No matter how you want to nurture and nourish your baby, it is important to decide before so that you will be able to prepare yourself. Whether breastfeeding, formula feeding, exclusively pumping, or a combination of any of those, they all have their benefits or disadvantages. Make sure you research which option will be best suited for you, and your family.

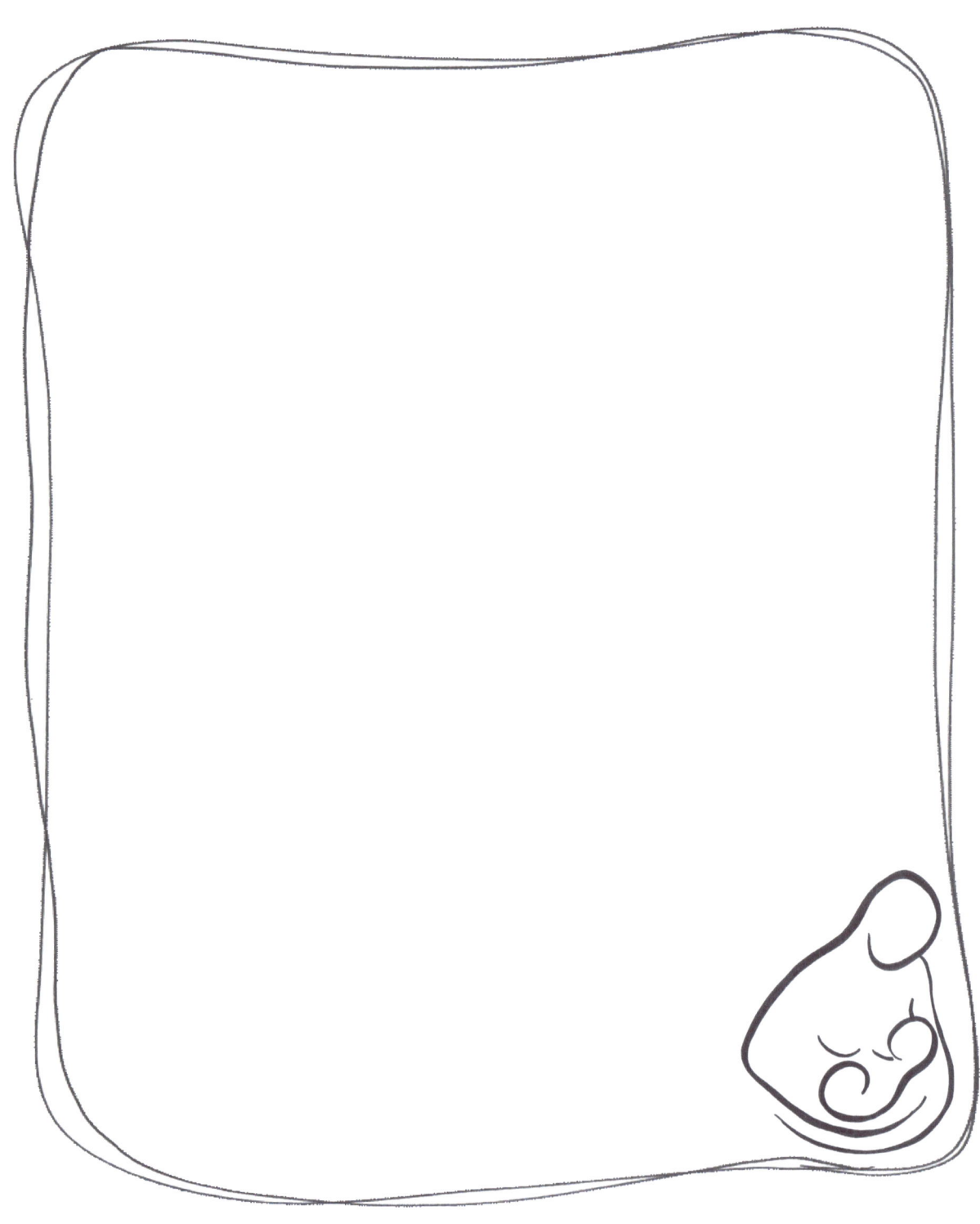

where will your baby sleep?

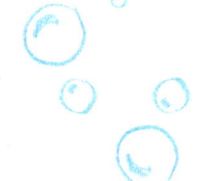

It is important to consider where your baby will sleep. The main options are co-sleeping (same bed, side car cot, or cot/bassinet in same room), or cot/bassinet in a different room. If you are considering co-sleeping in the same bed please ensure you do so safely. If either you or your partner smoke, drink, or are on medication that cause drowsiness it is not recommended to share a bed with an infant.

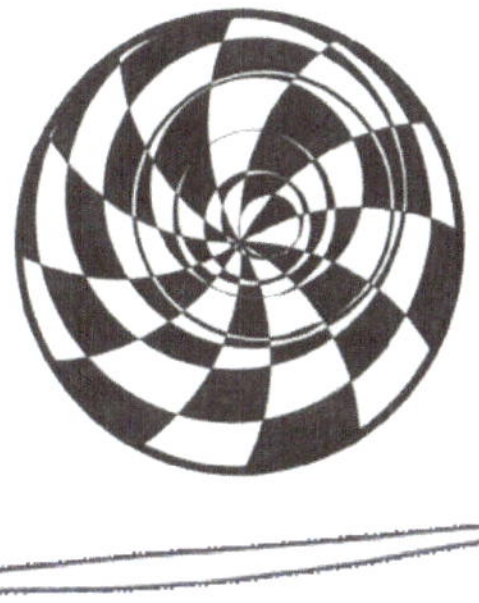

your Baby Moon

Immediately after the baby is born, there are many people who will want to share in the joy that is a new life. Have a think about the impact of an endless trail of visitors will have on you, your energy levels, and your ability to bond with your baby (and it with you). Ask people to help you after the birth, take some time to think about how that help will assist you the most. What jobs around the house would really help you out? What meals might people be able to cook for you to make it easier for you and your partner?

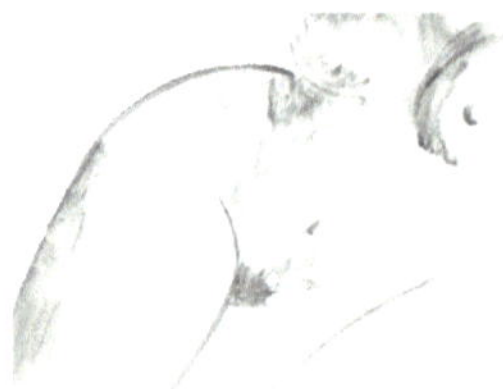

"When you change
the way you view birth,
the way you birth will change."

Marie Mongan

your Birth Story

This section is to be filled in after the birth of your baby. Take a week or two before writing it out, as it helps to have some time to process it, and to piece it all together afterwards.

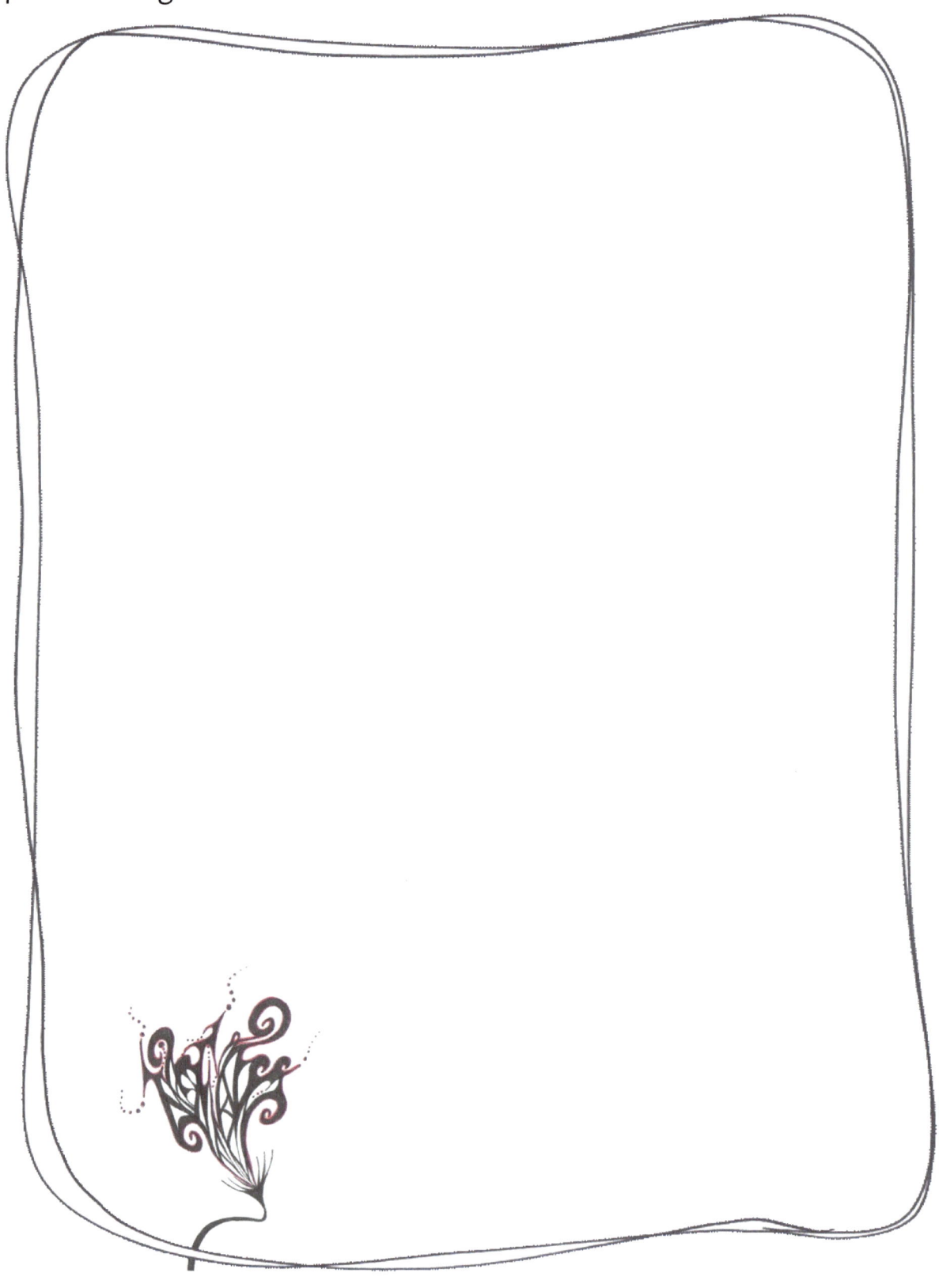

About April Wood

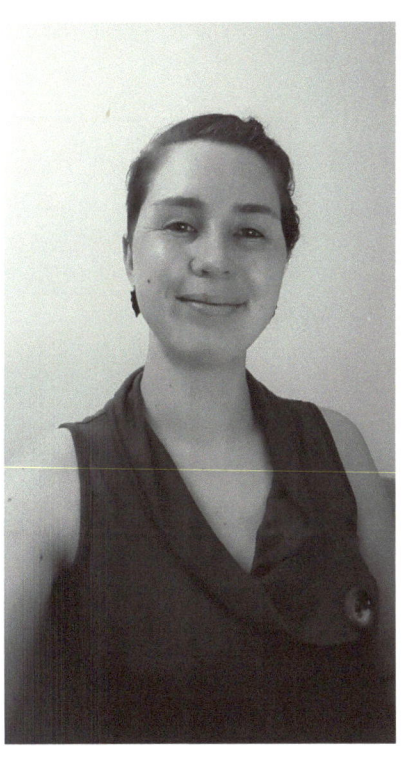

April is a woman of many talents including being
a qualified Acupuncturist, Breastfeeding Counsellor, Birth Doula, Postnatal Doula, Childbirth Educator, and trainer for other birth professionals. She is also a mother of four, an artist, and musician.

While working with her acupuncture and birth clients she recognised an increasing need for time out, along with thinking about where they were going, and
what was happening in their lives.

To fill this need April created a collection of books to help people to focus on
where they are at in their lives, and to take time out to rest their minds, while at the same time create beautiful artwork.

Visit her website www.nurturinglife.com.au to see what other books are also available.

Connect with me on Instagram:

@birthmandala or #birthmandala

www.ingramcontent.com/pod-product-compliance
Lightning Source LLC
Chambersburg PA
CBHW060808290526
45792CB00005BA/1570